Kratom

What You Need to Know

by Ryan Heffron

Table of Contents

Introduction

Congratulations on downloading Kratom: What You Need to Know.

Whether you came to find this book by curiosity or intent, I am glad you have joined me on this journey of discovering Kratom.

You may be wondering what is Kratom? What is it used for? Does it really benefit its users? How much can I take? Is Kratom even legal where I live? All very valid and common questions.

The intent of this book is to create a place where you, the reader, can find everything you would need, or want to know about Kratom, in one location. This book will be your guide as it takes you through the origins of this herb, its history, and discovery, to what it is today.

In the following chapters, we answer questions that you may have about Kratom. You'll read real stories from real people who have used this emerging plant and see through their eyes, an insight about the experience they had and let those who haven't taken Kratom, have an understanding of what this plant can do.

This book will provide you the information you need to hopefully create, a well-rounded view of Kratom. Whether you are for or against it, knowledge is the key to understanding. When you understand something you no longer have to feel afraid, instead you can be equipped.

So let's dive into this world of mitragyna speciosa... Kratom.

Chapter 1: What is Kratom

So what is Kratom? Sometimes Kratom is referred to by other names, such as kakuam, krathom, ithang, mambog or ketum depending on its region.

In the 1800's a Dutch settler discovered the plant in Thailand. Between 1839 and 1859, the tree was named and renamed several times. It was George Darby Haviland who finalized the name and classification: *Mitragyna speciosa*.

Is it a plant, tree, flower, animal? Kratom may sound like a scary sea monster of a mythical creation, but rest assured, it is not. Kratom is actually an evergreen tree that is a part of the Rubiaceae family, a species mostly known for coffee beans. This family is a large family, showing 630 genera and an estimated 13,000 species around the world. These plants aren't just ornamental, many are also used in folk medicine. About 60 species are used in 70 medical indications.

The mitragyna speciosa is typically found in tropical and sub-tropical environments in and around Southeast Asia. This area and its regions of Thailand, Malaysia, Indonesia, Myanmar, and Papua New Guinea are among the favored places to provide the perfect environment for these trees to thrive. The soil is wet humus and yet not too waterlogged. The proper pH for this plant is imperative, it must have a pH of 5.5 to 6.5 to survive.

Humidity is also a key player in its growth process. During the day in natural conditions, it's exposed to ninety-four percent humidity, at night the humidity is around fifty-three percent.

These trees can grow up to heights of eighty-two feet. Their leaves are dark green, broadly shaped like a mint leaf and glossy in appearance. The leaves can grow up to eight inches in length. The bold veins that run down the center of the leaves can be red, white or green in color. This color is significant in identifying the strain of plant.

Their trunks are greyish in color and smooth to the touch with flowers of yellow. The seeds from the mitragynine speciose are only viable within the first few hours to only a few days after departing the parent tree. These seeds are found inside a pod head, resembling a tiny spiked ball, and contains about fifty flat shaped seeds per pod.

Those who have tried to grow these plant at home find it difficult to keep the plant sustained. They require a very specific set of needs that are hard to facilitate in places away from its native origins. Though not unachievable, the price to curate this plant is far more expensive than it would be to just purchase the powder from vendors. The internet has created an open market for obtaining Kratom products readily.

The Rubiaceae/Mitragyna family.
There are several plants that are listed in this family, many are still yet to be classified and accepted as a genus of the Mitragyna strain.

Mitragyna diversifolia, Mitragyna hirsuta Havil, *Mitragyna inermis* (Willd.) Kuntze, *Mitragyna parvifolia* (Roxb.) Korth, *Mitragyna rotundifolia* <u>(Roxb.) Kuntze</u>, *Mitragyna tubulosa* (Arn.) Kuntze are all species that have some of the same properties that are seen in the mitragyna speciosa leaves but they pale in comparison to its relative. Not much is documented on these other species. A few details can be found for the M. Inermis, M. Javanica and M. Parvifolia species.

The M. Javanica strain appears to be the weakest on the scale. It does not share the same ingredient of mitragynine. This plant's primary compounds are mitrajavine and 3-isoajmalicine. Users of this plant say that the effects feel like a faint echo of what Kratom leaves induce.

M. Parvifolia was known as "kadamb." It's native to Northern India and does not grow to be the same height has Kratom trees do. This plant has different alkaloid properties such as dihydrocorynantheine, isorhynchophylline, hirsutine, and rhynchophylline. The effects of this plant is said by users to come on quick and last for very short periods of time, maybe 90 minutes or less. It is also said that it comes with jitters and a very unnatural nervous kind of energy. It can be found sometimes as the "Mellow Gold Strain."

The M. Inermis strain is said to be commonly used in traditional medices treating malaria. The main alkaloids in this plant appear to be uncarine D and isorhynchophilline.

Varieties of Kratom

There are several strains of Kratom. Most commonly known ones are red, white and green vein. Even though the stem is removed in the processing of the plant for consumption, the color of their stem is important to note. It will determine the effect it has on the induvial taking it, both physically and mentally.

Red Vein Strain

Most of the Kratom sold is of the Red Vein species. Its effects are known to be on the calming side. Physically, Red Vein reduces pain and sometimes is used to replace painkillers. The strongest form of Kratom can even be used to aid in opium withdrawal. There are several strains in the Red Vein family. Bali, Red Vein Thai, Red Vein Kali and Maeng Da are a few of the more common strains.

White Vein Strain

White Vein Kratom typically renders effects resulting in a positive mood, an energized feeling, better concentration and even considered an anti-depressant. Those who are sensitive to caffeine may find using White Vein strains to cause irritability or jitters. Some mix the variety of Red Vein and White Vein together to create a more balanced effect.

Green Vein Strain

Green Vein Kratom is viewed as a mix or middle ground between the Red Vein and the White Vein strains. Its effects are milder for both energy and pain relief. This strain is often used to combat social anxieties. When taken before going out, it can relax you and make you feel more engaged with those around. Some varieties of this strain are Green Borneo, Green Sumatra, Green Malaysian and Thai Green.

Yellow Vein Strain

This new strain is receiving high praises. It is found to be twenty percent more potent than the popular red strain, Maeng Da. Reports say that the effects of the yellow strain offer a more sophisticated feeling to the mind and body. It is said that this strain has no bitter taste, heightens visual perception, soothes the stomach, has swift symptoms and shows the best mind-clearing effects. Yellow Vietnam Kratom, Yellow Sumatra, and Yellow Bali are a few names of this strain. It should be noted however that there is no natural occurring yellow vein leaf. The process in which a green or white vein leaf is dried is altered to create this new yellow Kratom.

Chapter 2: Chemistry & Pharmacology

What's in Kratom leaves you may wonder? The main compounds found in these leaves are Mitragynine and 7-hydroxymitragynine. Kratom leaves contain at least 37 alkaloids but, about 60% of the alkaloid extraction from the leaves is mitragynine and around 2% is 7-hydroxymitragynine.

The chemical make-up

Let's take a closer look at these two main alkaloids found in Kratom.

Mitragynine:
The molecule formula: $C_{23}H_{30}N_2O_4$
Molecule weight: 398.50 g/mol

Mitragynine was first discovered by D. Hooper in 1907, later in 1921, a medical chemist by the name of Ellen Field, was the first known person to withdraw mitragynine from Kratom leaves and give this alkaloid its name. it wasn't til 1964 that the chemical structure was unraveled. The systematic name for this chemical is (αE,2S,3S,12bS)-3-ethyl-1,2,3,4,6,7,12,12b-octahydro-8-methoxy-α-(methoxymethylene)-indolo[2,3-a]quinolizine-2-acetic acid methyl ester. Other names its known by: 9-methoxycorynantheidine, (E)-16,17-didehydro-9,17-dimethoxy-17,18-seco-20α-yohimban-16-carboxylic acid methyl ester, , and SK&F 12711.

Mitragynine is the most abundant alkaloid present in leaves of the mitragyna speciosa plant. Structurally it's related to yohimbine but has a completely different pharmacology.

It is considered an opiate withdrawal suppressant and at low doses, mitragynine produces a yohimbine-like attachment to alpha-adrenergic receptors. At a high dosage, the attachment to the delta opioid receptors is increased. At very high doses, it will result in an attachment to the mu receptors, producing sedative effects. Chemically it is 9-methoxy-corynantheidine.

7-hydroxymitragynine:
The molecule formula:
Molecule weight: 414.50 g/mol

7-hydroxymitragynine is found in small amounts in the mitragyna speciosa leaves. This chemical was found later then mitragynine in 1993. The systematic name is:

(αE,2S,3S,7aS,12bS)-3-ethyl-1,2,3,4,6,7,7a,12b-octahydro-7a-hydroxy-8-methoxy-α-(methoxymethylene)-indolo[2,3-a]quinolizine-2-acetic acid methyl ester.

It is also an agonist and binds favorably to the Mu site at a value of 8.01+/-0.02. It interacts with three prominent opioid sites in the brain: Mu, Delta, and Kappa. It has analgesic effects and can have side effects of constipation.

Both mitragynine and 7-hydroxymitragynine are an agonist at the mu receptor. They bind and activate at less than 100 percent of the levels shown in other opioids such as morphine.

Chemical variances

The chemical make up in commercial products is varied and depends on many factors, the variety of the plant, the age, the environment of the plant, time of harvest, are all variables that change the potentness of the product. The alkaloid concentration in the dried leaves can range from 0.5 to 1.5 percent.

In Thai product varieties, mitragynine was found to be on the high side at 66% of the total alkaloids. 7-hydoxymitragynine was found to be about 2%. Malaysian products showed mitragynine at 12%, a much lower percentage of total alkaloids.
In Japan products, concentrated dried leaf or powered Kratom were found to have 12-21 mg/g and 0.11-0.39 mg/g. Resins showed 35.6-62.6 mg/g or mitragynine and 0.12-0.37 mg/g of 7-hydroxymitragynine.

Humans metabolize mitragynine by way of hydrolysis on the side-chain, O-demethylation of the methoxy groups, reductive and/or oxidative transformations, and the formation of sulfate and glucuronide conjugates. In one man who fatally overdosed on Kratom combined it with propylhexedrine. An autopsy revealed mitragynine concentrations ranging from 0.02 mg/kg to 1.20 mg/l.

Botanical alkaloid compositions can be analyzed by regular spectroscopic and chromatographic methods. Phylogenetic characterizations of Kratom can complement the phytochemical analyses.

Kratom alkaloids can be pulled apart by thin-layer chromatography (TLC) on a sheet of glass with detection by UV (254 nm). TLC is a technique of separating non-volatile mixtures. When Ehrlich's reagent or ferric chloride-perchloric acid reagent is sprayed on the specimen, the mitragynine shows up as purple or grey/ brown spots.

The UV spectrum of the methanol solution of mitragynine demonstrates a maximum at 225 nm with shoulders at 247, 285 and 293 nm. The infrared absorption bands found in the mitragynine are at 3 365, 1 690 and 1 640 cm^{-1} on the spectrum. Fragments in the electron impact ionization mass spectrum proved significant, (m/z): 398(M+), 383, 366,214,269,200 and 186.

7-hydroxymitragynine on the UV spectrum of ethanol solution showed a max of 220 nm with shoulders at 305 and 245 nm. The absorption bands found in the infrared spectrum for 7-hydroxymitragynine in chloroform, were at 3 590, 2 850, 2 820, 2 750, 1 700, 1 645, 1 630, 1 600, 1 490, 1 465 and 1 440 cm^{-1}. Fragments in the electron impact ionization mass spectrum proved significant, (m/z): 414(M+) 367, 383 and 397.

These alkaloids metabolites can be measured in the urine at >100 ng/ml by Gas chromatography-mass spectrometry, or GC-MS, this test is held as the "gold standard" in forensic substance identification. In the High-Performance Liquid Chromatography-UV or the HPLC-UV, test it shows up at >25ng/ml. For the HPLC-MS it shows up at >0.02 ng/ml.

For a better understanding, a forensic urine sample was taken from a regular Kratom user showing mitragynine concertation of 167 ng/ml using the HPLC-MS testing. In an autopsy of another individual that regularly ingested large doses of dried Kratom leaves, had a blood serum concentration level of 0.020 ng/ml of mitragynine, even after two weeks past the individuals passing.

Unveiling Kratom's potential

In 1960, Smith Kline French, later known as GlaxoSmithKline, wanted to replace the highly addictive drug, morphine, with the newly discovered mitragynine. Its properties after some testing were found to be close to that of codeine. At one point, they considered replacing codeine with the new mitragynine.

Christopher McCurdy, a medical chemist, and Boyer joined together in numerous studies. One experiment they embarked on was to see if Kratoms properties would prevent symptoms of opioid withdraw. They gave mice two doses of morphine every day, for five days. They doubled the dose every day until the mice were addicted. In a usual experiment, the mice would be given an opioid antagonist, like naloxone. The mice then would usually go through opiate withdraws. For this experiment, Mr. McCurdy and his colleague, gave the mice freeze-dried Kratom tea for five days before the mice would go through the opioid withdraw test. The results were significant. The mice showed a great reduction in side effects during their withdrawal, even more so then if methadone was used.

The National Institute of Thai Traditional Medicine in Bangkok, along with many other hospitals, recommend using Kratom in adding drug addiction withdrawals. Many reports have shown its success in helping patients free their bodies from the clutches of addiction. The common method in weaning heroin addicts is to prescribe methadone. The problem is, methadone has proven to be just as addictive as the substance the individuals were trying to be rid of. In some cases causes lifelong addictions. Kratom changes this whole process. Because Kratom renders short-term effects on the mu-receptors. Through a process of patience and time, addicts can free themselves with potential less adverse effects.

While some say Kratom could become addictive, others point out that it has no more addictiveness then caffeine.

Studies have occurred mostly on animals, but none have been done with humans much. A very extensive test was recently performed on ten human subjects. Several authors took part in writing this tests process and results. For the purpose of keeping the data in tack, the following report has been as closely relayed from the original as possible.

Authors of the following article are Trakulsrichai S, Sathirakul K, Auparakkitanon S, Krongvorakul J, Sueajai J, Noumjad N, Sukasem C, Wananukul W, Limsila P.

(https://www.dovepress.com/front_end/pharmac okinetics-of-mitragynine-in-man-peer-reviewed-fulltext-article-DDDT)

There were studies performed to observe the effect of mitragynine several years ago. The acute toxicities studied in rats include increasing blood pressure, hepatotoxicity, and nephrotoxicity. In another rat study, it was found that the aqueous extract, even very high dose, did not cause death and any significant toxicity. In humans, the adverse effects or the toxicities include dry mouth, changes in urination, nausea, vomiting, anorexia, weight loss, constipation, nystagmus, and tremor. In addition, seizure has been reported in previous literature. Primary hypothyroidism and intrahepatic cholestasis are also reported in a number of cases to be associated with Kratom. For chronic toxicity, impairment of cognitive behavioral function is found in mice fed mitragynine for a long period. In humans, anorexia, weight loss, hyperpigmentation, and psychosis are described in chronic abusers. Kratom alone, or in combination with other substances, has been shown to cause dependence and withdrawal symptoms following repeated consumption. Kratom has the potential herb-drug interaction on cytochrome P450 (CYP) enzyme activity. This was shown in one study, with potent inhibitory effect for CYP3A4 and CYP2D6, moderate effect for CYP1A2, and weak effect for CYP2C19, whereas in another study, mitragynine and 7-hydroxymitragynine also showed the inhibitory effect on P-glycoprotein. However, there were a few reports of Kratom-related fatalities.

To date, current knowledge of Kratom is limited, and many questions remain regarding its basic safety and the potential toxicities.

Hence, the pharmacology and pharmacokinetics are very important and necessary data to understand in managing poisoning or even widening the medical scope of Kratom in the future. Currently, the pharmacokinetics of Kratom has been derived only from animal studies, which employed only the rat model and produced variable results. There is no pharmacokinetic study in humans. Thus, the objective of this study was to look for the first time at the pharmacokinetics in humans and to assess the linearity of the pharmacokinetics of mitragynine, the most prevalent alkaloid in Kratom. This active alkaloid is a promising new chemical for new drug development.

The study was approved by Institutional Review Board of the Faculty of Medicine, Ramathibodi Hospital, Mahidol University.

Since Kratom is an illegal substance in Thailand, performing the study in healthy subjects is unethical; therefore, we performed the prospective experimental study in chronic regular users. We asked for permission to possess Kratom leaves from the Thai Food and Drug Administration to be used in this study.

The primary outcome was the pharmacokinetics of mitragynine. The secondary outcomes were blood pressure and pulse rate change after taking Kratom. We used different doses of Kratom to observe the dose responses in our study.

Inclusion criteria for recruiting subjects in this study included healthy participants, without any underlying diseases, using Kratom regularly for more than 6 months, having positive urine or blood test for mitragynine at the first hospital visit. We excluded subjects who refused to participate in the study. All subjects provided written informed consents.

<u>Study protocol.</u>

Preparation of Kratom tea

Kratom tea for this study was prepared from leaves collected from Pathumthani province, Thailand during 2012–2013. Ramathibodi Poison Center, Faculty of Medicine Ramathibodi Hospital was certified to handle the plant material. First, fresh or dried leaves of Kratom and different times for boiling the Kratom tea (30 minutes or 1 hour) were compared to find the most proper conditions. Fresh leaves and a 1-hour boiling time were selected for preparing the tea. In detail, 40 g of fresh Kratom leaves were cut and mixed together with 2 L of distilled water, and the leaves were boiled for 1 hour. Three mitragynine concentrations of tea were prepared: 0.1042, 0.166, and 0.1917 mg/mL. Then, the tea was kept in sterile 60 mL bottles and at 4°C for stability testing, which was performed at 3, 5, 7, and 14 days.

Prestudy period

On the first day, subjects were interviewed and underwent medical, physical, and basic psychological evaluations at Ramathibodi Hospital. The baseline mitragynine concentration and blood chemistry were also checked.

Since the subjects were chronic, regular users, and did not need to stop their Kratom use, we considered them adjusted to the steady state of Kratom levels by ingesting a known amount of Kratom tea (60 mL) every day for 7 days.

Study period

The pharmacokinetic study was performed on day 8. All subjects were admitted and resided in a ward for 24 hours. They were randomly assigned to take either 60 mL or

120 mL of the tea defined as loading doses or the 8th dose added in the study day. Forearm venous blood was collected from subjects through a heparin lock at 17 times points during the 24-hour period at time 0 (before the loading dose was given), 15, 30, and 45 minutes; 1, 1.25, 1.5, 1.75, 2, 2.5, 3, 4, 6, 9, 12, 19, and 24 hours. Urine samples were collected during the period of study to measure Kratom concentrations.

For physiologic changes and safety, vital signs, as well as any abnormal signs and symptoms, were also observed during the study period.

Specimen analysis

Chemicals

Mitragynine was purchased from Cerilliant Corporation (Round Rock, Texas, USA), 7-methyltestosterone from Fluka Chemie GmBH (Buchs, Switzerland), ethyl acetate from Thermo Fisher Scientific (Waltham, MA, USA), and acetic acid and methanol were from Merck KGaA (Darmstadt, Germany). All chemicals were of analytical grade.

Analysis of plasma and urine samples

A 0.5 mL aliquot of each subject's plasma and urine samples (indicate period of collection) was spiked with 25 µL of 2.0 µg/mL 7-methyltestosterone (internal standard) to achieve final concentration 100 ng/mL. A 2 mL aliquot of 0.1 M phosphate buffer, pH 6.0, was added and briefly mixed. The solid phase extraction (SPE) column (C18; Agilent Technologies, Santa Clara, CA, USA) was conditioned with 2 mL of methanol and a 2 mL aliquot of 0.1 M phosphate buffer, pH 6.0. The plasma or urine sample then was loaded onto a conditioned SPE column, and 1 mL of deionized water and 1 mL of 10 mM acetic acid were added to the SPE column, which was dried for 5 minutes under vacuum (<20 mmHg). Analytes were eluted with 3 mL of ethyl acetate and dried under a flow of nitrogen gas below 40°C. This residue was reconstituted with 100 µL of 20% acetonitrile.

Analysis of Kratom tea

A 10 µL aliquot was added to 990 µL of 20% (v/v) acetonitrile, mixed, and centrifuged at 13,800× g for 5 minutes at room temperature. The supernatant was used for subsequent analysis.

Liquid chromatography-tandem mass spectrometry analysis

The sample volume of 5 µL (for plasma or urine) or 2 µL (of Kratom tea) were analyzed using an Amazon SL LC-MS/MS system. Liquid chromatography was performed in an UltiMate 3000 UHPLC system (Thermo Fisher Scientific) equipped with a Luna-C18 separation column (100 mm ×2.1 mm; 3 µm particle size) and the same phase guard column (10 mm ×2.1 mm; 3 µm particle size). All samples were kept at 10°C in autosampler trays during the analysis cycle. Mobile phase A was composed of 5 mM ammonium acetate together with 0.1% formic acid, and mobile phase B was acetonitrile with 0.1% formic acid. After the introduction of the sample, the mobile phase was initiated at 10% B (90% A) and linearly increased to 40% B within 10 minutes, then to 75% B within 13.5 minutes, and finally to 80% B within 16 minutes and maintained for 5 minutes.

Mass spectrometry was performed in an amaZon SL Ion Trap spectrometer (Bruker Daltonics, GmbH, Germany). A standard electrospray ionization source was operated in positive ion mode with the nebulizer at a gas flow rate of 8.0 L/minute and drying temperature of 250°C. End plate offset and capillary voltage was 500 V and 4,500 V, respectively. Multiple reaction monitoring transitions was 399.20→238.20 and 303.20→285.20 for mitragynine (retention time 9.10 minutes) and 7-methyltestosterone (retention time 13.74 minutes), respectively. Line spectra were collected in full scan mode from 50 to 1,000 Da. The validation of the analytical method was performed and will be published separately (Auparakkitanon, unpublished, 2015).

Pharmacokinetics and statistical analysis

The pharmacokinetics of mitragynine was evaluated by use of computer software, WinNonlin® version 3.0 (Pharsight Corporation, Mountain View, CA, USA). Noncompartmental analysis included determination of the following parameters: the maximum or peak plasma concentration (C_{max}); the time to maximum observed concentration or time to reach C_{max} (t_{max}); terminal half-life ($t_{1/2}$), estimated via linear regression of time and the log terminal end portion of the curve; and the area under the time-concentration curve from the time of dosing to the time of the last observable concentration ($AUC_{0-tlast}$), calculated by the log-linear trapezoidal rule. The area under the curve (AUC) extrapolated to time to infinity ($AUC_{0-\infty}$) can be calculated by adding $AUC_{0-tlast}$ with the last observable concentration (C_{last}) divided by linear regression-fitted terminal slope (λ_z). The apparent total clearance (CL/F) was calculated by dose/$AUC_{0-\infty}$. The apparent volume of distribution (Vd/F) values were calculated in L/kg of body weight and were computed based on the terminal elimination phase and the apparent CL/F. Data were reported as the mean ± standard deviation (SD) unless otherwise defined. Repeated measures ANOVA were tested for continuous data of mean blood pressure, pulse rate, and capillary blood glucose. The mean and SD were for continuous data, and the frequency and percentage were for categorical data.

Results

There were ten subjects recruited in this study. All were healthy men who had no preexisting diseases. The demographic data is shown in Table 1. The liver and kidney function values were within an acceptable limit.

Table 1

The demographic data of ten subjects

Characteristics	Frequency
Sex, Male (%)	10 (100)
Age (year), mean ± SD	27.1±4.7
Weight (kg), mean ± SD	77.3±14.8
Height (cm), mean ± SD	170.8±7.2
Body mass index (kg/m^2), mean ± SD	26.4±3.9
Duration of abuse (year), median (min–max)	1.75 (0.6–5)
Kratom leaves consumed/day, median (min–max)	4 (1–9)

The data from our laboratory analysis showed that mitragynine concentration in the tea was stable during storage at the subjects' homes, and this meant that the subjects actually received the same dose every day.

The daily doses and loading doses were different and divided into five groups, as shown in Table 2. The normal and semilogarithmic plot of plasma mitragynine concentration against time curve of every subject after the administration of a loading dose is shown in Figure 1. We found the abnormal behavior of blood concentration in one subject, which was clearly far different from that of the other subjects. This subject's parameter was analyzed separately. The highest C_{max}, 0.105 µg/mL, and the highest $AUC_{0-tlast}$, 0.67 µg h/mL, were found in the subject taking the highest loading dose, 23 mg. The lowest C_{max} was 0.0185 µg/mL, found in the subject with the low loading dose 9.96 mg. The lowest $AUC_{0-tlast}$ was 0.062 µg h/mL, found in the subject with the lowest loading dose, 6.25 mg. The T_{max} was 0.83±0.35 hours and the average apparent Vd/F and CL/F of mitragynine were 38.04±24.32 L/kg and 98.1±51.34 L/h kg, respectively, as shown in Table 3. The semilog plot of pharmacokinetics time profiles in nine out of all ten subjects demonstrated biexponential decline, which suggested the pharmacokinetic behavior of mitragynine followed the oral two-compartment model, as shown in Figure 1. The correlation between the loading dose and C_{max}, as well as the loading dose and $AUC_{0-\infty}$, were linear (Figures 2 and 3). When the dose increased, the C_{max} and $AUC_{0-\infty}$ increased proportionally with dose. We found that the CL/F was quite constant and not increased when the loading dose increased. Altogether, it was suggested that the pharmacokinetics of mitragynine was linear or first order kinetics. The urine excretion of unchanged mitragynine was very limited, as it was only 0.14%.

Figure 1:

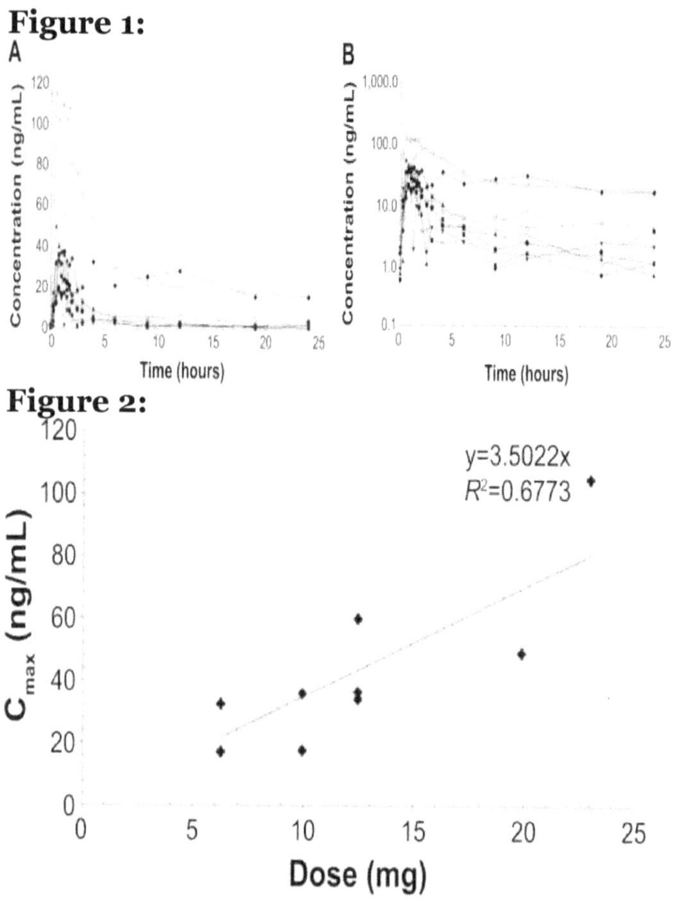

Figure 2:

Figure 3:

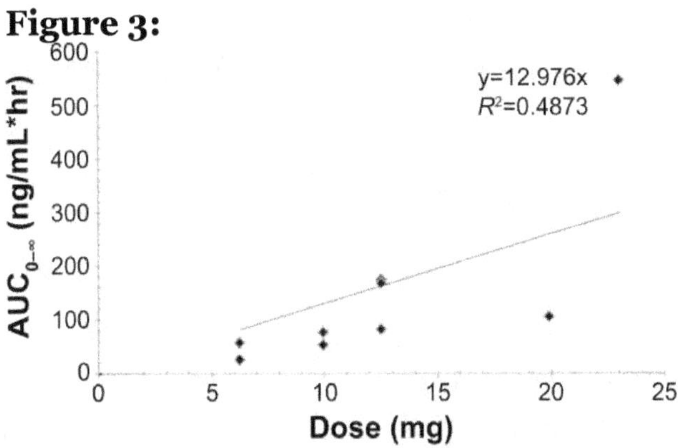

Table 2:

The number of subjects, the daily mitragynine doses to adjust for the steady state, and the loading doses in each subject

Daily dose for 7 days (mg/day)	Loading dose (mg) in the study day (8th day)	Number of subjects
6.25	12.5	3
6.25	6.25	2
9.96	19.92	1
9.96	9.96	3
11.5	23	1

Table 3:

The summary of the pharmacokinetic parameters of mitragynine

Parameters	Mean ± SD
T_{max}(h)	0.83±0.35
Terminal $t_{1/2}$ (h)	23.24±16.07
Vd/F (L/kg)	38.04±24.32
CL/F (L/h kg)	98.1±51.34

Abbreviations: CL/F, clearance; SD, standard deviation; $t_{1/2}$, half-life; T_{max}, time to reach the maximum plasma concentration; Vd/F, volume of distribution; h, hour.

For one subject who took 9.96 mg for both daily and loading doses and had the abnormal behavior of blood concentration, his normal and semilogarithmic plots are shown in Figure 4. There was no distribution phase because no sharp decrease in the blood concentration was seen. The possible errors were excluded by reevaluation. His blood samples were collected for other investigation in this regard.

The blood pressure and pulse rate of every subject increased at the 8th hour of study and then returned to normal, as shown in Figure 5 and 6. Capillary blood glucose levels were normal during the period of the study. All subjects described tongue numbness after they finished drinking Kratom tea. No abnormal signs and symptoms were detected during this period of the study.

Figure 5:

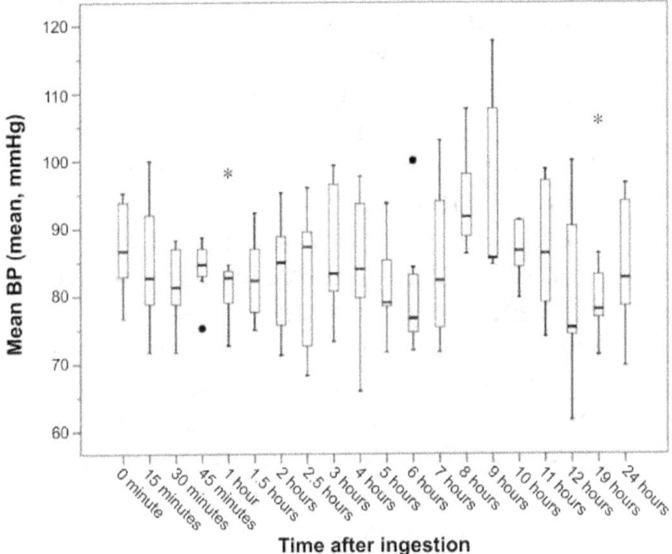

Figure 6:

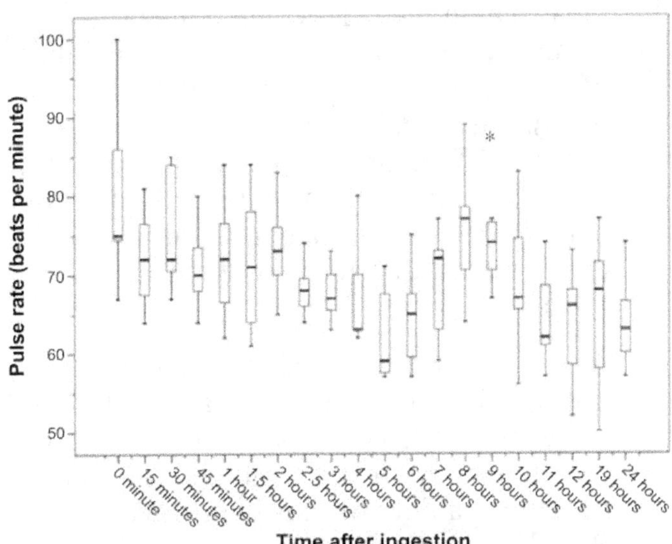

Discussion

The pharmacokinetic parameters are important and essential information for the pharmacologic study of any substance of interest. To our knowledge, this study was the first pharmacokinetic study of Kratom in human. In our study, the pharmacokinetic parameters were different from those of animal studies. As we used different doses, more information was added, showing the pharmacokinetics were linear and followed an oral two-compartment model. Information on the bioavailability of oral mitragynine is not currently available in humans. The Vd and CL in our study were apparent Vd and CL. According to this apparent Vd, it would be considered as a large Vd, unless the bioavailability was less than 2%. For example, we applied the oral bioavailability of mitragynine from the rat study, which was 3.03±1.47% in our pharmacokinetic analysis. The estimated Vd and CL would be 1.15 L/kg and 2.97 L/h kg, respectively. We hypothesize that mitragynine has a large Vd and is mainly distributed out of the circulation.

As urine excretion of the unchanged mitragynine form was as low as 0.14%, this suggests that renal excretion should not be a significant route of excretion, even when its bioavailability was taken into account. Based on our findings, we propose that mitragynine is mainly metabolized by hepatic metabolism to other metabolites. This is consistent with another study on mitragynine.

As for the clinical and safety aspects, no serious adverse effect was found during the study. This is probably because the doses used in our study were less than 30 mg. However, the daily intake dose of regular abusers was reported to be as high as 276.5 mg in Malaysia. Every subject in our study developed tongue numbness after having finished drinking Kratom tea. All of the participants also confirmed that it was the same experience as when they took Kratom. Thus, tongue numbness would be one of the symptoms of Kratom effect that was supported by these studies.

Our study also found that all subjects had increased blood pressure and heart rate, but the onset was delayed to 8 hours after drinking Kratom tea. The time was later than T_{max}; therefore, this finding needs further investigation.

For clinical applications, the beneficial effects of Kratom on opioid withdrawal have been reported in various studies. Our study showed that it had a long elimination $t_{1/2}$ and linear pharmacokinetics. Taken together, Kratom would be a good candidate for opioid substitute in patients who are addicted to these substances. As it had very low renal clearance, in patients with impaired renal function, dose adjustment might not be needed.

However, based on the finding that the pharmacokinetics of mitragynine is linear, if dose adjustment is needed, it can be easily implemented. Extracorporeal techniques such as hemodialysis or hemoperfusion might not be able to remove mitragynine from the circulation as it would have high Vd/F.

In conclusion, pharmacokinetics of mitragynine, a major and active metabolite of Kratom, is linear and follows the two-compartment model. It has a long terminal $t_{1/2}$, extending for hours, and high apparent Vd. Renal excretion of unchanged mitragynine is very low. The pharmacokinetics of Kratom in human was different from animals, thus applying the animal data to humans should be used with caution. Numbness of tongue would be a clinical marker of Kratom ingestion. Abnormal pharmacokinetics in some patients and delayed onset of increasing blood pressure and heart rate require further investigation.

Kratom has been an emerging substance of abuse, available worldwide. In the future, Kratom may merit further scientific study to develop its medical benefits, as a better opioid substitute, with fewer lethal side effects, or as an effective painkiller.

Drug tests

Drug testing and finding abnormalities in the body are always improving. To that end, some have had results come back and show a false positive for Methadone and subsequently effecting their job or pursuit of a job. The amount of Kratom taken may have been a player in those individuals drug test producing the false negative. Many over the counter medications can show similar results on a drug test.

Other users, however, say that Kratom does not show positive on drug tests. Their reason, it does not have the same opiate metabolites and does not show up on the tests. In recreational users of Kratom, mitragynine concentrations can be found in levels between 10-50 µg/L.

As the alkaloids are broken down and metabolized in the liver, the breakdown product is released in the urine, saliva, and blood. Elimination timeframes are varied from half-life of one day to half-life of six days."

Chapter 3: Legality of Kratom

Kratom currently is still viewed as a psychotropic plant that resembles other substances of opiate classifications and is seen as potentially addictive. In 2013, it was placed on the ASEAN list and cannot be used in traditional medicines and health supplements that are traded in the ASEAN nations.

The Association of the Southeast Asian Nations, or ASEAN, was formed on August 8, 1967, by the countries Thailand, Indonesia, Malaysia, Philippines, and Singapore. Its membership has grown to include Cambodia, Brunei, Laos, Vietnam, and Myanmar. Its main purpose and function are to promote social progress, economic growth and sociocultural evolution among its members as well as protection of regional stability and provide a mechanism for member countries to resolve differences peacefully.

ASEAN is an official United Nations observer and active global partner. Its territorial reach is about three percent of the total land mass on earth. The territorial water coverage is three times larger than its land mass coverage. The combined population of its membership countries is about 640 million people or 8.8% of the world's population.

It's a good idea to check your current laws where you live before you using Kratom, as the laws about its legality can and do change. Kratom is currently legal in most countries. However, it is illegal or banned in Australia, Finland, Malaysia, Myanmar, and Thailand.

Thailand

Kratom is ironically illegal in its native country, Thailand.

In 1920, the Thailand government saw that the plant grew in abundance throughout the country. Because of this, it was being sold for a very cheap price on the market and could often be found for free. It was then that the government saw that they weren't getting as much as they wanted from their opium trades and thus in 1943, the Kratom Act 2486, which prohibited the indigenous trees from being planted, was placed into action.

Kratom is now classified in Thailand in the same category as heroin and cocaine. Punishment for having even an ounce of the extract is death. Some will use a species closely related to the mitragynine speciousa, *Mitragyna javanica,* however it is considered not as effective. In 2004, 2009 and 2013, Thailand did consider legalizing Kratom.

An article written by Keith Cleversley in 2013, gives us an understanding of Thailand's history and sheds some light on why Kratom is banned in its indigenous region today. (http://entheology.com/news-articles/why-kratom-was-banned-in-thailand/)

> "... The 1930's and the 1940's were a
> tumultuous time in Thailand on many

levels. They were marked by a military dictatorship that bludgeoned the citizens of Thailand from the 1930's up to the 1970's. The military came to power in the bloodless Siamese revolution of 1932, which transformed the government of Siam (Thailand) from an absolute to a constitutional monarchy. The new regime of 1932 produced a constitution in December of 1932, which was Siam's first. It included a National Assembly, that promised that full democratic elections sometime in the 1940s.

By 1939, political unrest had reached a pinnacle. In that year, forty political opponents, both monarchists and democrats, were arrested, and after rigged trials eighteen were executed, the first political executions in Siam in over a century. Many others were exiled. The government launched a campaign against the Chinese business class, closing anything Chinese, while taxes were raised to alarming levels. A man named Luang Phibunsongkhram was in power during this time.

Phibun used the exact propaganda techniques that were used by Hitler and Mussolini o build political power. Aware of the power of mass media, the government's monopoly on radio broadcasting was also used to shape popular support for the regime. During this time, Phibun passed a

number of authoritarian laws which gave
the government the power of almost
unlimited arrest and complete press
censorship.

Seething within the underbelly of this
political turmoil was the ever-present black
market. Not surprisingly, one of the largest
black market trades was the opium
trade. Knowing how profitable it was, the
Thai government passed a series of laws
that levied duties and taxes from every
aspect of the opium trade that they could;
from the grower, to the manufacturer, to
the distributor, to the shop owner and even
the end consumer. It was a "cash cow" for
the government.

With this boom in opium consumption,
there was also a boom in opium addicts,
opium-related deaths, and general public
health concerns that come with any drug,
licit or illicit. The government was clearly
in the opium trade, as it was profiting
heavily from it. With the amount of money
that was generated from their taxes and
levies, this was an aspect of money
generation that was worth protecting.

Well, in the fields of Thailand, where
workers often toiled in the fields for 16-18
hours a day, often with no days off, there
was an amazing plant that helped them get
through their days. This plant was known
as Kratom (Mitragyna speciosa). Not only

did it help mitigate the pain they felt from all of the hard physical labor, it provided them with a mild sense of calm, of peace, to help them get through their day.

In fact, Kratom was often referred to the "poor man's marijuana", as it became associated with field workers who couldn't afford the more expensive Cannabis that was widely available. From a few pieces of literature I've found on the subject, if a man was asking for a woman's hand in marriage, he was held in higher regard if he was a "Kratom chewer" rather than a "Cannabis smoker". That meant he was a hard worker, dedicated to family values, and not afraid of work in general.

Kratom spread like wildfire across the working class people of Thailand, and they were using this widely-available, often-free, safe, non-addicting, natural plant instead of opium. In fact, what was even more alarming to those with conflicting interests, is that many of these new opium addicts who provided easy and reliable income to the government, were finding respite from their addictions by using Kratom to alleviate their symptoms.
In other words, as early as the 1930's, the people of Thailand had discovered that Kratom was a powerful means of helping them with their opium addictions. Not only did Kratom tress grow everywhere in Thailand, it was easy to boil down a few

leaves, and make a "Kratom Ball"; the most common form of ingestion of this plant at the time.

War broke out in 1942; the East Asian War as history has called it. When war breaks out, it's terrible for the economy, and all of the taxes from the opium trade that the government had enjoyed suddenly vaporized. The government raced to find ways of bringing back the cash cow they had enjoyed as a result of the opium trade. One of the first things they did, was look to see if there was any competition in this particular market.
Sure enough, Kratom, which had swept the nation, and was accompanied by little to no adverse reactions or hospital visits of any kind (unlike opium), was now seen as a threat to the massive amounts of cash bring brought in because of the opium trade.
Kratom was one of the "low hanging" fruits, and easy target:

A member of the House of Representatives from Lampang in a special meeting on 7 January 1943 (Police Major General Pin Amornwisaisoradej) said this: "Taxes for opium are high while kratom is currently not being taxed. With the increase of those taxes, people are starting to use kratom instead and this has had a visible impact on our government's

income."

An act was passed called "The Kratom Act", which criminalized Kratom. By now, its use was so widespread (it had been part of Thailand culture for over 3,000 years), that anyone in the working class was at least familiar with Kratom, had a friend, family member, or even relied on its safe, effective use themselves. Kratom tress were grown with impunity, the millions of acres of naturally-occurring Kratom trees flourished, and leaves were chewed openly in public without any fear of arrest. So, it seems that the Kratom Act was never really enforced.

Fast forward to 1979:
In 1979, kratom was included in the "Thai Narcotics Act", under Schedule 5 (the least restrictive and punitive level). It was added to the same classification that Cannabis and psilocybin mushrooms belonged to. The Kratom Act had severe penalties for ingesting Kratom, and this was intended to reduce the sentences and the punishment for those found to be in violation of the Kratom Act.

So, although Kratom is still criminalized in its home country, it's at least on a level with other mis-categorized natural herbal products, which allows for the possibility of a policy change that would finally place Kratom back where it belongs; as a safe, effective herbal supplement that has a wide range of medical benefits…"

Malaysia

In Malaysia, Kratom is locally called "ketum," and many are petitioning their government to do research on Kratom as a medicinal purposed herb. However, in January of 2007, Malaysia has made strides to make it more illegal in their country, rather than less. The country plans to classify it under their dangerous drugs law instead of, the less severe, poisonous substances law. People found using Kratom may be fined a maximum of 10,000 MYR ($3,150 USD) or be put in prison for up to four years.

Australia and New Zealand

In January of 2015, Australia controlled the substance and now views it as a narcotic. Its decision to banned Kratom seems to have been based on a few influences. One being that Kratom's native country has banned its use and a study paid for by Smith Kline, a pharmaceutical manufacturer. The study may have been a push for pharmaceutical motivations seeing as how Kratom is an all-natural herbal remedy, which means less business for the pharmaceutical industry.

New Zealand's policy can be easily misunderstood. An individual can buy Kratom but they must have a prescription. Possession of the herb without one is considered illegal.

Canada

Canada does not permit Kratom to be ingested and
is considered illegal in that form. They do however
allow it for other uses, such as incense. Any
company marketing Kratom in a digestive form
will have actions taken against them.

The United States of America

The United States has, as of August 2016, placed
Kratom on the Schedule I of the Controlled
Substances Act.

Schedule I substances are usually described as
1. Drug or substance has s high potential for
    abuse
2. Drug or substance is not currently accepted
    as medical use treatment in the United
    States.
3. Level of safety is lacking for drug or
    substance under medical supervision.

Prescriptions cannot be written for Schedule I
substances.

Kratom was being marketed as a dietary
supplement but the FDA has not approved
mitragyna speciosa for human consumption. In
order for a herb, supplement or novel food to be
approved by the FDA requires a substantial
amount of capital and a lengthy trial process. It
can cost upward of $50 million USD and take
several years before a decision is reached.

For this reason, packaging now cannot provide instructions on how to safely use the product. With the lack of information and guidance is puts individuals at risk of taking higher doses then would be ideal, possibly developing tolerance.

Vendors can advertise Kratom legally if it's labeled as ethnobotanical for collection purposes, research herb or as incense. FDA rules can't control what a buyer does with the substances. Which means the buyer can choose how to use the product without fearing legal ramifications.

There is a divide on Kratom. Some have not had good encounters with the substance and others praise its abilities to help deal with pain, weaning from opioids and alcohol. Later in May of 2016, Alabama, Arkansas, Indiana, Tennessee, Vermont, and Wisconsin all have made Kratom illegal in their states.

1,175 doctors, vets, scientists and law officers in the US, told the DEA they did not want to see Kratom banned.

Europe
In 2011, the plant was controlled in Denmark, Lithuania, Latvia, Poland, Romania, and Sweden. More recently in the United Kingdom, the sale, export, and import of Kratom were prohibited under the Psychoactive Substances Act.

Finland

Some reports say that Finland allows the use of Kratom but requires a prescription to buy it. The plant itself, if tried to be imported, would be seized at the border.

Hungary

The leaves are not approved for human consumption but it can be found and bought in head shops as incense.

Myanmar or Burma

It's illegal to grow or sell the herb.

Romania

As of 2010, Romania as banned the substance in its country.

South Korea

Kratom is illegal in this country and has heavy penalties for possession of any kind. Penalization will be that of criminal punishment.

Sweden

There are some indications that the laws may change in the future but currently, it is illegal to use.

Chapter 4: Benefits and Potential Healing Properties

Kratom traditional uses
Traditionally Kratom was used by peasant workers to help them have more energy and relieve their aches and pain after a long hard day working the fields.

As a medical value, it was used to treat mild problems. Fever, diarrhea, diabetes and as a poultice for pain.

There are four African and six Asian Mitragyna species that are known to be used in traditional medicines. Only the Mitragyna speciosa has the narcotic/stimulate/sedative like characteristics. In the Southeast Asia region it is used an antidiabetic, antidiarrheal, deworming agent, and cough suppressant.

Some benefits you may already be aware of such as increased energy, improved mood and an overall better sense of well-being. But let's take a closer look at these areas.

Pain Reliever
Kratom leaves have a rich analgesic property and can quickly relieve pain in the body by targeting the hormonal system. Serotonin and dopamine are increased in your bodies release when you chew the leaves. The pain receptors are dulled throughout as the alkaloids are released.

Immune System
Some studies have shown that Kratom leaves can have effects of strengthening and adding resilience to the immune system. The leaves are equipped with free radical scavenging and antimicrobial activity that are a natural source of antioxidants.

Increased energy
Increase in energy is the most popular feature of these leaves. The alkaloids optimize certain metabolic processes and target your hormone levels. The results are an increase in circulation and a general increase in oxygen to the body, combine this with the metabolic activities and you have a burst of energy. Those who have Chronic Fatigue Syndrome use Kratom leaves as a natural alternative solution.

Increased libido
In many traditional practices, users of Kratom have used it as an aphrodisiac and a fertility booster. The extra energy and blood flow stimulated by the leaves can help increase fertility, re-energize the libido, and improve duration.

Anxiety reducer
By regulating the hormones in the body, people can find relief from the exhausting symptoms and chemical imbalance of chronic stress, depression, anxiety and mood swings. Not having to rely on pharmaceuticals and the side effects it brings is praise enough for some users.

Addiction Recovery

Because the nature of Kratom leaves is such a combination of effects, it has been used in methods of curing addictions for hundreds of years. Opium addictions are found in many cultures and when the leaf of the Kratom plant is chewed, people who are seeking to "get clean," can do so without having to endure such negative side effects when coming off addictions.

A testament to Kratom addiction release

One person's personal testimony with Kratom, will truly just show how much it can benefit and bring healing to people's lives.

Jason, a hardworking man, worked physically taxing jobs most of his life and in the process caused damage to his back. His first-hand account of how Kratom became a part of his life, freeing him from the grips of addiction, will hopefully show the potentials of this amazing plant.

> "I've worked rather hard my whole life, I've done everything from hanging drywall to landscaping so as you can imagine, I was pretty rough on my body growing up.

> Back in 2005, I had enough of the pain I was constantly in and went in for some pain management. The doctor that treated me diagnosed me with chronic lower back pain that also came with painful muscle spasms. Eventually, I was pretty dependent on 180+mg of morphine a day. The Addiction

that came with it was out of control,
absolutely horrible.

I am also a medical marijuana patient now
too, but at the time of my crazy addiction, I
had failed a drug test for THC. I was
instantly cut off of my pain medication, I, of
course, had my remaining prescription, but
knew I had to do something. I believe I was
actually looking for an internet Doctor
when I first read the word Kratom. Through
more surfing, I eventually looked into more
information about the stuff. I finally just
tried Kratom. I was absolutely amazed at
the fact that it really managed my pain and
spasms. The best part about Kratom is that
my addiction to pills just kind of went away.
I never felt like I "Needed" opiates again.
My stress and anxiety are even better.

I take Kratom religiously... twice a day every
day now. I pretty much vowed to introduce
this god given herb to everyone I possibly
can. I have, and probably always will see
people struggle with pain, and addiction to
pain medications, and I'll be the first one to
hand out some Kratom. If I can potentially
save lives, even just help someone in need...
You Bet I Will! I am living proof of the
positive change this tree can make in
someone's life."

Chapter 5: Consumption methods, dosages, subjective effects

The traditional use of Kratom was to chew the leaves, rendering pain relief, increased energy, sexual desire, and appetite. They were used to heal wounds and were useful as a local anesthetic. Diarrhea, coughs and intestinal infections were also treated by the Kratom leaf and its extracts.

In its native country of Thailand, it was used as a snack when guests came over and were part of a ritual to their ancestors and gods.

Kratom and its forms

Figuring out what dosage amount is right for you and your needs can be difficult but highly important. Dosage is based on strain type, tolerance levels, body type, desired effect and concentration levels.

Kratom can most commonly be found as a powder. They can be used in capsules, teas and even as an incense. The leaves themselves can even be chewed as in the traditional method. It's been mentioned one could smoke the substance, however, there is not much proof to show effects can be felt by using this method.

Generally, you would take Kratom on an empty stomach to maximize its efficacy. Its bitter taste usually has individuals mixing it with a sweetener for easier consumption. If taken in capsule form the effects can be delayed. Taking anywhere between sixty to ninety minutes before the full effect is reached. The higher the dosage the stronger the effects and potential longer effectiveness.

There are a few methods that people recommend when consuming Kratom powder. As the taste is bitter and difficult for some to ingest on its own,

Mixing with a drink.
It's suggested to mix the powder with a beverage. Most often orange juice is good at masking the tastes of the powder. Some also brew a tea, served either hot or cold.

Mix with food.
Some find mixing the Kratom powder in food to be a fun, flavorful combination. There are some recipes that show how to incorporate the powder into your food. The sky can be the limit on how you cook with it. The flavor combination and balancing of how much powder will of the chefs making.

Extracts and Enhanced Kratom
The majority of Kratom products are a raw, unprocessed leaf that is ground into a fine powder.

An extract has become steadily popular of the years, as they are stronger than the regular leaf. The process of making an extract is done by boiling a large amount of leaves from the mitragyna speciosa tree, down and compressing it into a small smooth rock, known as resin. This resin is then ground into a new "extract powder." Extracts can be up to twenty times more potent than in its original form.

Enhanced Kratom is a combination of the extract with regular unprocessed leaf powder. It's considered a middle ground between the regular strength and super strength options.

There does exist a level of Kratom known as "Ultra Enhanced."

When this is seen on the label for Kratom it is cautioned and is not intended for the novice user. These products deliver a very high potent experience.
Ultra-Enhanced or UE can be up to 1500 additional milligrams of pure alkaloids.
Typically this ultra-enhanced powder is made by boiling down the resin, made from the first time to make the enhanced resin. Dosages for this product will be significantly smaller than the other less potent products.

This option is more expensive but users say you use less so it may balance out in the cost factor with using unprocessed Kratom powder.

Super or Premium

You may find that some products have the words "super" or Premium" along with the strain of Kratom on the packaging. These added words specify the way the leaf is processed and render a bit more concertation then the usual powder.

Super, indicates the specific production technique. When the plants are harvested, the larger leaves, or super-sized leaves, are used for this blend as they hold more bioactive alkaloids and result in a higher concentration. Rendering the powder made from these leaves, a higher quality product.

Premium, is referring to the harvesting method of the leaves. In this process, the stems during harvest are carefully removed from the leaves before it is ground into powder. Giving the consumer a good balance between high quality and reasonable pricing.

Dosages

If you were to look at a scale of what Kratom usage could look like, this scale shows the mild stimulant state to heavy stimulated state in grams. Every user has a different tolerance level but in general, it could look something like the following:

1-2 grams; little, to no feeling.
3-5 grams; become slightly more focused
6-10 grams; you'll feel as if you've caught your second wind and feel very happy
11-15 grams; physical pain and anxiety will start to fade
16-25 grams; strong effects, even euphoric at times.

25+ grams; very strong effects, usually too strong to handle.

In the low dose range of 1 to 5 grams, you may experience:
- Decrease appetite.
- Increased energy.
- Increased alertness.
- Increased social ability.
- Increased libido.

In the moderate to high dose range of 5 to 15 grams, you may experience:
- Pain reduction.
- Drowsiness.
- Dreamlike mental state of being.
- Cough suppression.
- Reduction of symptoms from opioid withdrawal.

In the high dose range of 15 grams and greater, you may experience:
- Extreme sedation.
- Loss of consciousness.

The different strains and their effects

The different strains of the mitragynine specious will deliver varied results.

If you were to consume Bali, for example, a Red Vein strain, the effects general are for relaxing, pain killing and reducing insomnia. Usually, the effects start to make themselves known between twenty to forty minutes. Its duration can be up to five hours.

The Green Vein strains effects are mostly for mood lifting, concentration, and subtle stimulation. The onset of the effects will again be around twenty to forty minutes and can last up to eight hours.

The White Vein strains deliver high energy, better productivity and lifting depression. It will take effect in the twenty to forty minute time frame. This strain will last up to three to five hours.

The New Yellow Vietnam strain is compared to the Red Vein but with a more sophisticated touch.

Here is a list of some strains, their effects, and dosage amounts.

Strain	Effects	Dosage
Bali	Euphoric. Most common of Kratom strains.	.5 to 3 teaspoons
Maeng Da	Energizing with painkiller effects	.5 to 3 teaspoons
Red Vein Thai	Similar to Bali with less negative side effects	.5 to 3 teaspoons
Red Vein Kali	Sedating. More of an opiate.	.5 to 3 teaspoons
Green Vein Kali	Stimulating with painkiller effects	.5 to 3 teaspoons

White Vein Thai	Stimulating, Euphoric and dissociating effects	.5 to 3 teaspoons
Super Green Malaysian	Stimulating with little euphoria	.5 to 3 teaspoons

Frequent Kratom users are recommended to rotate the strains to reduce any risk of addiction. In general, it's a good practice to not use the same Kratom multiple days in a row. Rotating strains means your body will not build up too rapidly of a tolerance and thus slowing down this process and providing a wider scope of alkaloids.

Enhanced or UEI dosages

Enhanced high-quality Indo Kratom is effective with only a single gram, about one-eighth of a teaspoon, of powder. Often time's users prefer half of this dosage at .5 grams

Tolerance

Our bodies have a way of adapting to regular behaviors and building tolerance levels to many things. So how can you identify if your body is has become tolerant? Dosage amounts that you previously used do not render any effects, causing you to have to increase your dosage amount. Increasing the dosage amount will mean an increase in side effects.

One way to prevent your body from becoming tolerant of Kratom is to follow a few simple guidelines when you use it.

- No re-dosing in a day. One session or dose is pretty adequate for users
- Limit back-to-back. Allow at least one day between usage.
- Keep the same dosage. Once you find what works for you, try not to increase it on your next session.
- Sample a range of products. Try to alter the strain you use, or try a different region where the strain is grown.
- Do not overuse the enhanced products. This will increase you tolerance levels faster as they are highly potent blends.

So, what does it feel like?

You may be wondering what these "effects" really feel like. How does this actually effect your body?

Everyone's physical and mental state is affected differently. Some may experience little effects with a low dose while other may be highly sensitive. Finding the right amount and balance will take practice and is recommended to start small, gradually increasing the amount over time.

As a general guide, the following may be experienced:

At the stimulant level: Your mind will be more alert. Physical energy and sometimes sexual energy is increased. Many times you will feel more social, talkative and outgoing.

At the sedative/euphoric/analgesic level: You are less aware of physical or emotional pain. You feel a scene of calm and can enter the mixed state of "waking-dreaming." You can experience some nausea but lying down usually will solve this issue. Your pupil may constrict (become smaller) and you could feel sweaty and itchy. Some have said they had a positive afterglow the following day.

A personal experience

One user's experience using the Maeong Da, was described as a two- tier process.

At the first tier, there is a burst of energy similar to a strong cup of coffee. The energy from Kratom was longer lasting and more steady then caffeine derived energy. The energy level from Kratom was subtle, lasted for three to four hours and they did not experience any energy crash, unlike caffeine.

The second tier was a relaxing effect. It was not a sleepy form of relaxing but rather a feeling of being balanced from the energy burst first experienced in tier one.

This user did not experience any side effects worth much mentioning. They said their eyes seemed a bit bloodshot at times but wasn't a consistent side effect. It did not affect their vision.

As for the withdrawal process. After stopping the use of Kratom, for this induvial, there was little to no effect. Sluggishness was experienced but wore off after a few days. This same individual shared when they come off coffee they experience extreme headaches and anger for at least two days.

The overall comment on Kratom by this user is that it was like a good cup of coffee, but with a better "finish."

Chapter 6: Toxicity and Abuse

Some have wondered if overdosing on Kratom is possible. There is a bit of confusion on this. While the leaves contain opiate compounds, it's also believed there are opiate antagonists that overrule or dominant the mitragynine and 7-hydroxymitragynine as the dosage increases. This is where you will feel symptoms of nausea or vomiting. It would be difficult or nearly impossible, to consume an amount high enough to overdose. The side effects alone would be very unpleasant in trying to consume more.

Are there side effects?

Side effects are a possibility. Kratom's effects vary from person to person. Some people may not experience any side effects, while others have reported short-term effects of nausea, itching, sweating, dry mouth, constipation, increased urination, loss of appetite, weight loss, anorexia, and insomnia. Some long-term effects reported have been insomnia, darkened skin, and anorexia. The most cautioned side effect is the addiction possibilities.

Those who are heavy users of Kratom could experience withdrawal symptoms such as a runny nose, muscle and joint pain, diarrhea, nausea, hypertension.

Respiratory depression is another concern. Kratom affects the mu-opioid receptors, and in animal studies, a very high dose of mitragynine caused respiratory depression. A study of Kratom and its chemical effects has not been studied in people yet.

So... is Kratom addictive?

Advocates for Kratom argue there is little risk of becoming habit forming or dangerous if it's used responsibly. Like all things, moderation is key.

However, some individuals who may have addictive personalities or addictive tendencies may find occasional use difficult and it could become habit-forming.

Long-term users may build up tolerance levels and have to increasingly up their dosage to get the same effects. There was a study done that showed fifty percent of those who used Kratom regularly for 6 months showed dependency. The dependents suffered similar physical withdrawal symptoms to those of opiate users.

The Center for Disease Control or CDC

The US CDC found that abuse of Kratom leads to irritability, agitation, tachycardia, nausea, hypertension, and drowsiness. Other health risks found were psychosis, seizures, hepatotoxicity, insomnia, tachycardia, weight loss, vomiting, poor concentration, hallucinations and even death were reported.

There are some who will combine Kratom with other substances, this practice is cautioned against as Kratom on its own is potent enough. Combining substances in a dangerous mix and can lead to very serious health risk or even death. One dangerous mixture is known as Krypton. This concoction is a mix of Kratom and O-desmethltramadol. These two ingredients combined increase the depressive effects on the central nervous system and have been known to cause death.

Toxicity of Kratom

Toxicity on a serious level is rare and generally only seen when a high dosage of Kratom, 15 grams or greater, was used with other substances.

Liver toxicity is still in question. In a rare case of chronic usage of Kratom, acute liver injury was reported, accompanied by fatigue, itching, nausea, and jaundice.
Cholestasis is associated with liver injury. Cholestasis is a condition where bile, a fluid produced by the liver, cannot pass from the liver to the duodenum (the first section of the small intestine).

Interestingly, no reports of toxicity or death due to Kratom have been reported in the Southeast Asia area. It is not known if this is because the users are able to tolerate Kratom more due to its history of use in the area, or simply because any reactions just go unreported. The only report known as of current was in Thailand, but it was later found that the user had mixed Kratom with other illicit drugs, like codeine.

It is speculated that the leaf being consumed in Southeast Asia is unprocessed and leaves being used in the West are a stronger, more potent blend that may have other substances in the power.

Kratom has shown in test to be toxic to animals.

Chapter 7: Success Stories and the Future of Kratom

Is there a place for Kratom? There are many individuals who have discovered Kratom at a point when they thought all was lost. What they experienced ended up saving their lives. One such story is from an induvial that suffered both mental and physical pain.

A testimony that saved a life

"When I was about 20 years old I got braces on my crooked teeth to straighten them out. Every month I would go back to my Orthodontist & he would change the wires on the braces & tighten them a little bit each time to bring my teeth a little straighter each month. So each month for about a week my teeth would really hurt me & my Orthodontist would not prescribe me any pain meds because he didn't have a License to write any prescriptions.

I tried all the OTC pain meds but nothing worked. I was in agony for about a week. That's when I started getting opioid pills & pretty soon I was hooked on them just about a week. I just wanted more & more. I wore those braces for about 2 years until I had to have them removed to have an MRI of my head because I was having very bad Migraine Headaches every week but the scan turned out to be normal.

I also had Severe Chronic Depression since I was about 15 years old & I tried a dozen different prescription anti-depressants & none of them worked but when I started taking the Opioids I noticed that my depression was completely gone for about 3 hours & then back to my depression & back to my teeth hurting again. So far about 5 years I was addicted to any kind of pills that I could get my hands on to make my depression feel better or just to get high.

I went to 3 Outpatient Rehabs & that kept me clean for a little while but then after a month or so I was back to using again. I must have stopped on my own about a dozen different times but each time I would start back using again within a week or two later. I overdosed 3 times, had 3 car wrecks & hurt many family members & many close friends with my addiction.

My addiction was totally in control of my Life back then. My worst overdose was when I passed out & I was rushed to the ER & my Oxygen Level was only about 80%. It's supposed to be above 95% I think. I was very close to dying then.

I tried other Herbs & Botanicals & nothing would help my Depression or addiction. I also was diagnosed with Mild Autism when I was about 27. I also have Social Anxiety Disorder, Obsessive Compulsive Disorder, Agoraphobia, Migraine Headaches, Under-active Thyroid Gland & many other minor health problems.

Then when I was about 25 I found this herb called Kratom (Mitragyna Speciosa). Once I started taking it every day my life completely turned around. I no longer had depression, had no urge to take any opiates to get high. Kratom just made me feel like life was worth living again. I was more social & had less anxiety. My migraine headaches were much better. Everything that I did wasn't like going through the motions in life but Kratom made the little things enjoyable again instead of dreading the day-to-day things that we do every day to survive in life. If I didn't have Kratom I would have died years ago on pills.

Kratom helps with so many different aspects of my life now. It helps me socialize whenever I get out of the house, calms my anxiety, takes away any pain that I may have, my depression has been gone for 7 years now since I've been taking it, helps me with insomnia when I can't get to sleep. I love to talk about anything to do with Kratom. I've learned so much over these 7 years that I've been taking it daily. It has never failed to work for me. It has never made me sick with any bad side effects. It is a great antioxidant with numerous benefits that no other herb or botanical can hold a candle to. Nothing compares to Kratom. Kratom could help so many millions of people with their addictions to any drugs or alcohol. It also can help with withdrawals when getting off of any drugs or alcohol.

To me, Kratom is the most valuable herb on the planet. It has so many benefits that no other medicine can match. Nothing comes close. There are so many different strains of Kratom that can produce different desired effects. Kratom is a very intricate plant. You don't just take it & it produces the same desired effects every time. You can vary the dosage, mix different strains, consume it different ways or take it in different forms & each will produce a different very unique desired effect.

It affects each person a little differently so you will have to learn all about it & experiment about which strains & what dosages are best for you. I only take Plain Leaf Kratom. I stay away from any enhanced or extracts. I highly recommend only taking Kratom in Plain Leaf Powder Form & nothing else. I just hope they keep this amazingly wonderful plant legal for all of us to benefit from.

What is Kratom's future?

There are hundreds of success stories out there to suggest there is not only a need for Kratom but a necessity for it. When used responsibly, the benefits can far out weight the negative.

With further research and time, it is possible to show its potential. There so much more about this plant and its abilities we still don't know.

Conclusion

Thank you for reading *Kratom: What You Need to Know*. Hopefully, you found this book informative and able to provide you with all of the tools you need to achieve your goals whatever they may be.

With more time and research, Kratom has so many faucets still yet to be discovered. It has the potential to unlock a whole new world of information. There are so many alkaloids still unknown within this plant, who knows what could come of looking further into its unlocked doors.

If you found this book useful in any way, a review on Amazon is always appreciated!